Essential Oils For Diffuser:
40 Delicious Essential Oils Blends For Your Home

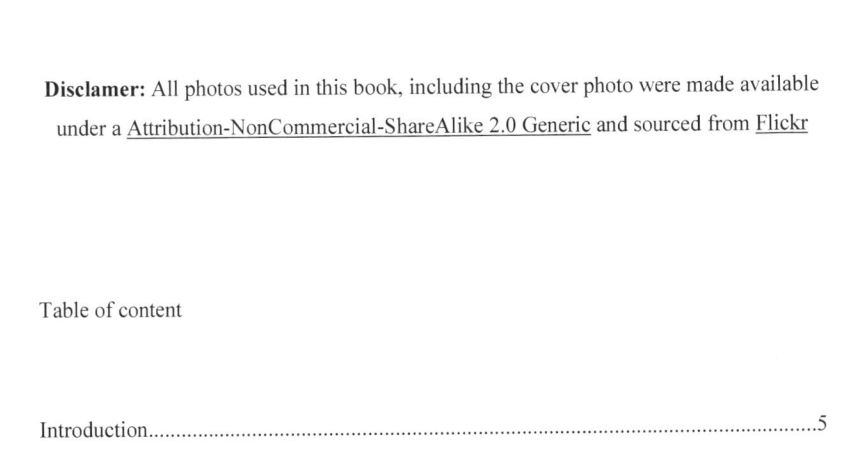

Disclamer: All photos used in this book, including the cover photo were made available under a Attribution-NonCommercial-ShareAlike 2.0 Generic and sourced from Flickr

Table of content

Introduction..5

Facts About Essential Oils 6

Caution! 8

Facts About Essential Oils to Keep in Mind 8

Keep Essential Oils Away from Your Pets! 9

How Long Does Essential Oils Usually Last? 10

What Do You Want to Use Essential Oils for? 11

Benefits of Using Essential Oils 12

Diffuser Types and What they Do 12

Essential Oil Diffuser Recipes 13

1. Spirit Uplifting Blend 13

2. Flowery Flow Blend 13

3. Nice & Spicy Cider Blend 14

4. Feeling A Little Under the Weather Blend 14

5. Wintergreen Winter Blend 15

6. Holiday Time Blend 15

7. Refreshing Your Carpet Blend 16

8. Refreshing Body Mist Blend 16

9. Out Musty Smells Blend 17

10. Cedarwood Scent for Clothing Blend 17

11. Inhaling Stress Reliever Blend 18

12. Relieve Aching Feet Blend 19

13. Wake Up! Blend 19

14. No More Feeling Down Blend 20

15. Killing Nasty Odors Blend 20

16. Bright, Light & Fresh Blend 21

17. All-Seasons Blend 21

18. Citrus Mist Blend 22

19. Breath Better Blend 22
20. Bedtime Blend 23
21. The Guys Blend 23
22. Stop and Sniff the Flowery Blend 24
23. Joyful Blend 24
24. Keep Those Nasty Bugs Away Blend 25
25. Nite Nite Blend 25
26. Getting A Boost Blend 26
27. Peaceful Bliss Blend 26
28. Looking Lively Blend 27
29. Cheery Breaths Blend 27
30. The Healing Blend 28
31. Relaxed Breathing Blend 28
32. Leaving the Worry Behind Blend 29
33. Exercise Boost Blend 29
34. Feeling Frisky Blend 30
35. Tuned In Blend 30
36. Calm Blend 31
37. Keeping Allergies at Bay Blend 31
38. Citrus Garden Blend 32
39. A Little Ray of Sunshine Blend 32
40. Easy Breathing Blend 33
Conclusion 34

Introduction

I would like to first thank and congratulate you on downloading **Essential Oils: 40 Refreshing and Sweet Diffuser Recipes."** Many of the adult population deal with headaches at least once a year, this is a common disorder of the nervous system. When a person suffers from a headache it can really cause them to have a painful disruption to their day, causing them to be unable to continue with their daily plans. There is a large number of headache suffers that have come to find relief of their painful headaches by using a diffuser.

Often people will try an assortment of synthetic drugs that often are accompanied with bad side effects. I hope that you and your loved ones will be able to find some great peace and relief when using this collection of diffuser recipes that I have put together for you. Just think how nice it will be to finally get rid of that headache without resorting to synthetic drugs!

In order to make use of the diffuser recipes that I have provided here for you—you will need to invest in a diffuser before you can begin to enjoy the diffuser recipes supplied here in my book. I can honestly say that there is certainly no shortage of diffusers to choose from you will have a large assortment of different types that you will be able to choose your personal style of diffuser. The four basic categories of diffusers that you will have to choose from are heat, evaporative, ultrasonic and nebulizing. I will briefly describe each of these types of diffusers in the book—under the "Facts About Essential Oils" section. I hope that you will enjoy and benefit from the diffuser recipes that I have collected for you within this book!

Facts About Essential Oils

Looking back into our history we can trace the use of essential oils back to the Egyptians as being the first people to make use of essential oils in their beauty treatments, food preparation, health purposes, as well as cultural and religious activities. Essential oils were often exchanged by the Egyptians for gold, sandalwood, cinnamon, myrrh, and Frankincense as these items were much sought after back in this point in time.

A French chemist, Rene-Maurice Gattefosse, in 1937, during modern times, discovered the great healing powers that essential oils possessed. At the time he was tending to a patient who had bad burns, he added lavender oil to the patient's burns to help heal his burnt hand. Later a French contemporary, Dr Jean Valnet, gained fame due to his developments in using aromatherapy practices. He introduced aromatherapy to injured soldiers during World War II. Researchers and medical practitioners have had a large influence on the growing industry surrounding the use of essential oils in regards to health and wellness benefits that we can gain from their use with the proper application.

There are many countries throughout the world that include essential oils in their therapeutic aromatherapy, Ayurvedic, and massage purposes as well. Essential oils during the 'Dark Ages' were mainly used for their fragrant and anti-bacterial properties. Essential oils are sought by people worldwide that believe that they have healing agents within them. Many people are using them within remedies that will help treat ailments from skin conditions to cancer. There has been much popularity gained in the branch of alternative medicine better known as aromatherapy with essential oil playing a vital role in this form of treatment. Using the aromatic plant extracts they are used in treatments and cosmetic purposes.

Around the world there is some countries that have imposed regulations for the use of essential oils, it is still popular in being used for natural remedies and fringe medicine. There is researchers that are making the claims that essential oils have the ability to prevent the transmission of certain strains of pathogen, specifically Candida, Streptoco, and Staphylococcus that are drug resistant strains.

You may use essential oils for many purposes, applying them as a single oil or have them be used as part of a complex blend of oils. There are three different methods on how you are able to distribute essential oils: applied topically, diffused aromatically, or taken internally as dietary supplements which you should have these recommended by a physician.

Caution!

You need to be aware that there is many different kinds of essential oils that if taken by mouth due to their high concentration could cause a person to feeling a burning sensation followed by salivation.

One of the first things you should learn is never to apply undiluted essential oils to your body as it could cause or create sensitization. You could end up causing a bad skin rash, or even in extreme cases going into anaphylactic shock or respiratory issues occurring. If you find that you have an allergic reaction to an essential oil you may become permanently sensitized to that particular oil, even if you have diluted it. If you are unsure of the dosage of essential oil to use then seek out the guidance from a person that specializes in working with essential oils such as an aromatherapist or do some research online to find some answers to these questions.

Facts About Essential Oils to Keep in Mind
- Never apply any essential oils on or around your eyes or open wounds or sores. Do not use essential oils if you are pregnant or have epilepsy or asthma.

- Do a small skin patch test to assure that you are not allergic to an essential oil before you spread it all over your body.

- Make sure that you are buying 100% Therapeutic grade essential oils, read labels on how to store it properly.

- Always dilute essential oils in a carrier oil before you apply them to your skin. There may be exceptions to this rule—these should only be made by aromatherapy practitioners, not a novice.

- Keep your essential oils in a safe and appropriate place, store them like you would any other medicines in your home.

- Essential oils are flammable—keep out of reach of children and pets!

- Never take essential oils internally unless you have been prescribed to do so by a professional that specializes in the distribution of essential oils such as an aromatherapist.

Keep Essential Oils Away from Your Pets!
You might have read that it is okay to use essential oils as a form of treatment against such things as ticks and fleas. Using essential oils are highly safe for us humans to use but they can be highly toxic to our beloved pets. Essential oils such as Thyme, Lavender, and Terpenes can actually cause liver or kidney failure in cats. To be safe please do not attempt to use essential oils on your pets. It has been discovered that Tansy is poisonous to horses and cattle. Look for signs if your pet may have encountered accidental exposure. If your animal is showing signs of distress you might need to get them to the vet to be checked out. I had essential oil on my arm which my tongue licked she was fine—but let us not take a chance with the health of our pets if we do not have to.

There is still great debate on the use of using aromatherapy internally. The use of essential oils being used internally is discouraged by the National Association of Holistic Aromatherapy.

In traditional medicine essential oils are becoming more and more relevant as scientists are discovering that the fundamental materials do possess a value due to their wide array of components. In modern medicine they are leaning more towards holistic approaches to wellness looking into a new discovery of essential oil well-being applications for the future.

You can help safeguard yourself from contracting certain ailments such as colds by taking different Eucalyptus essential oils to help protect you against catching a dreaded cold by building up your protection barrier. By choosing the right essential oil to diffuse you can change your mood just by the fragrance that emanates from the diffused essential oil. I would also suggest that you stay away from using Plugin air fresheners. These contain harmful chemicals and can cause damage when inhaled. Choose a much healthier and safe choice and choose an essential oil diffuser for your home.

Get creative and place a vase of dried lavender beside your headboard, it will help calm you and aide you in falling into a nice relaxing sleep.

How Long Does Essential Oils Usually Last?
There is multiple factors with regards to the shelf life of essential oils. If for example something occurs to cause the oils to destabilize this will result in the deterioration being sped up. The temperature, sunlight and atmosphere around the essential oils will have an effect on them, even when you keep them in the best conditions. Some oils could last you a lifetime when others may deteriorate rather quickly. Make sure when you are purchasing oils buy a therapeutic grade being 100% pure essential oils. Observe what the storage conditions are of the product you are purchasing. When the oils are kept in proper storage containers this is going to help ensure they are preserved and will offer you the greatest level

of impact. When storing oils you should keep them in a dark, cool place, making sure that there is no influence of weather or temperature effecting them.

Many people are intrigued with essential oils but do not know the proper ways to apply them. The easiest way and safest way you can benefit from the use of essential oils is to disperse them using a diffuser. When you diffuse essential oils into your home environment you will add anti-bacterial and antiviral actions into your air supply; these will help destroy and ruin microbes in the air within your home. If you use a diffuser for antiviral/antimicrobial activity and immune support you can disinfect the air supply of your home. You can use a nebulizing diffuser that can help cut down the costs so you can evaporate therapeutic doses of essential oils into your home environment that will benefit you greatly.

What Do You Want to Use Essential Oils for?

If you are just searching for an essential oil that will make your home smell nice then you can choose a cheaper grade or food grade that is not very expensive. These types are often distilled using synthetic solvents and do not contain any pure essential oils. It is highly unlikely that they are 100% pure for a lower grade of essential oils.

The lower grades of essential oils do not carry with them any kind of therapeutic values. The lower grade essential oils you can purchase in many shops. If you are looking to use essential oils as part of a therapeutic remedy then you need to use a therapeutic 100% pure grade of essential oils. These grades of oils will carry solvents and come tested meeting the required standards to be classed as 100% pure essential oils. These grades of oils are expensive and are only supplied by a few quality suppliers.

Look for a supplier that has a good name for supplying quality therapeutic essential oils. You can do some research to find out who are the best suppliers near you for quality grade 100% pure therapeutic essential oils.

Benefits of Using Essential Oils
Some of the benefits you will gain from using essential oils are the following:

- You will find that you have a feeling of peace and calm.
- It can be a great way for you to boost your immune system.
- It can help reduce the stress in your life and improve your mood.
- It will leave your home smelling so wonderful!

Diffuser Types and What they Do
Diffusers basically break up the essential oils into little particles then they diffuse them into the air or your household environment. It is best for you to choose good high grade essential oils, you do not want to be inhaling anything that has other chemicals mixed into it. If you go with 100% pure grade therapeutic essential oils then you know you are making the right and healthiest choice. You will of course have a wide selection of diffuser to choose from. When you inhale the essential oils from the air they are going to go straight to your brain and other parts of your body as well, with the brain regulating and moderating all of your body functions.

There are four different main categories of diffusers: ultrasonic, nebulizing, heat and evaporative. Some of the common carrier oils used with essential oils are grape seed oil, sweet almond oil and olive oil. I hope you will enjoy the essential oil diffuser recipes and will use them to your benefit!

Essential Oil Diffuser Recipes

1. Spirit Uplifting Blend
Ingredients:

- five drops of Citrus Fresh
- one drop of Juniper
- five drops of Myrrh
- eight drops of Hinoki

Instructions:

Blend your oils and diffuse into the room and wait to feel your spirits being uplifted!

2. Flowery Flow Blend
Ingredients:

- 20 drops of Jasmine
- 20 drops of Royal Hawaiian Sandalwood
- five drops of Frankincense
- five drops of Balsam Fir

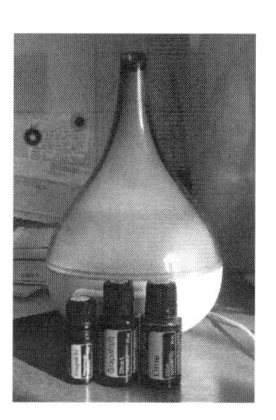

Instructions:

Once you have blended your oils and diffused them enjoy this wonderful flowery smell that will flow through your home. You will feel like you are taking a stroll through a flower garden!

3. Nice & Spicy Cider Blend
Ingredients:

- five drops of Orange
- five drops of Cinnamon
- four drops of Ginger

Instructions:

This spicy blend will help you to become nice and calm feeling grounded and ready to take on the world. Just blend and diffuse and feel the calm!

4. Feeling A Little Under the Weather Blend
Ingredients:

- four drops of Frankincense
- four drops of OnGuard Blend
- three drops of Lemon

Instructions:

This blend of oils is what you want to diffuse in helping get rid of the nasty germs in your home environment and will also boost your mood while it fights the germs!

5. Wintergreen Winter Blend
Ingredients:

- four drops of White Fir
- four drops of Cedarwood
- two drops of Cypress
- four drops of Wintergreen

Instructions:

The aroma you will get from this lovely blend will have you thinking you are out walking amongst nature!

6. Holiday Time Blend
Ingredients:

- four drops of Cassia
- two drops of Orange
- two drops of lemon

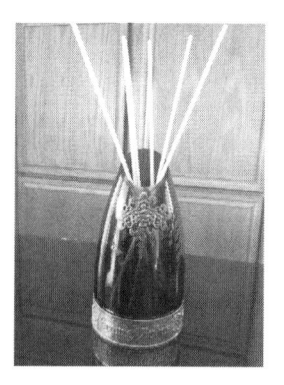

Instructions:

You will find that your spirits will be lifted with this blend during the special holiday times.

7. Refreshing Your Carpet Blend
Ingredients:

- one cup of baking soda
- three teaspoons of Lime
- one Teaspoon of Tangerine
- one quarter of a teaspoon of Litsea Cubeba

Instructions:

Take a mason jar and mix all of the ingredients into it and let sit for overnight. Then you can take this mix and sprinkle it on top of your carpets. Leave on for half and hour and then vacuum it up. Humidity can cause carpets to smell, it could be full of bacteria and mold. Adding this great carpet freshener will make your carpets smell great. Keep any that you do not use in an airtight container in the fridge.

8. Refreshing Body Mist Blend
Ingredients:

- two ounces of unscented base body mist or spray
- five drops of Vanilla Absolute Pure
- 10 drops of S'Woods
- 25 drops of Coconut Emulsifier

- four drops of Litsea Cubeba

Instructions:

Combine your oils in a two-ounce PET bottle adding the emulsifier to the bottle. Add into it the two-ounces of unscented body mist. Shake this well and spray it on your body after you have had a bath or shower.

9. Out Musty Smells Blend
Ingredients:

- ten drops of lavender
- twelve drops of Cedarwood
- twelve drops of Lemon
- six drops of Lime
- two teaspoons of coconut emulsifier

Instructions:

Add all of your oils along with your emulsifier, fifty-drops for half a teaspoon of emulsifier. Add all to PET spray bottle adding four ounces of water and shake the contents very well to mix. Spray on top of surfaces that you are getting a moldy smell from.

10. Cedarwood Scent for Clothing Blend
Ingredients:

- 35 drops of Cedarwood
- 12 drops of Clove bud
- 16 drops of Orange

Instructions:

Use an amber or dark colored bottle to blend mix in. You can add about several drops of this blend to a Terra Cotta Disc Diffuser. Wait for the oil to soak into the Terra Cotta Disk then place in are where clothing is kept. You will soon find that your clothing is left with a lovely Cedarwood scent.

11. Inhaling Stress Reliever Blend
Ingredients:

- four drops of Lime
- two drops of Lemon
- five drops of Rosemary
- five drops of Basil

Instructions:

Once you have blended your oil mix add to a cotton ball and put into a plastic bag. Then inhale this aroma nice and deeply. You will gain focus and will keep your mind open to the tasks at hand.

12. Relieve Aching Feet Blend
Ingredients:

- three drops of Spruce needle
- one tablespoon of Epsom salts
- three drops of Tea Tree oil

Instructions:

When you are having a nice foot soak add about two or three drops of this blend to the foot bath.

13. Wake Up! Blend
Ingredients:

- three drops of Peppermint
- one drop of Lemongrass
- two drops of Lime
- two drops of Orange

Instructions:

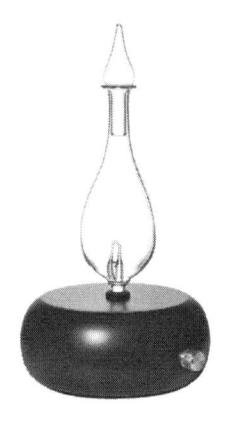

This blend is great in helping you to feel much more on the ball and wide awake and ready to start your day! This blend would work really well in a cold-air diffuser adding small amount of water and blending then you can diffuse and feel yourself come to life!

14. No More Feeling Down Blend
Ingredients:

- three drops of Geranium
- three drops of Melissa
- one drop of Sandalwood
- two drops of Basil

Instructions:

Inhale the depression out of your life with this wonderful blend that will have you no longer feeling down but up and in good spirits.

15. Killing Nasty Odors Blend
Ingredients:

- three drops of Lemon
- two drops of Melaleuca
- three drops of Lime
- two drops of Cilantro
- two drops of White Fir

Instructions:

All you have to do is blend your oils and diffuse them, they will attack nasty odors in your home and have your home environment smelling fresh and clean in no time.

16. Bright, Light & Fresh Blend
Ingredients:

- four drops of Lavender
- three drops of Lemongrass
- three drops of Rosemary

Instructions:

This great blend of oils will make the atmosphere of your home environment one of peace with a light and bright air to it!

17. All-Seasons Blend
Ingredients:

- three drops of Lavender
- four drops of Peppermint
- two drops of Lemongrass

Instructions:

You will find that this blend works

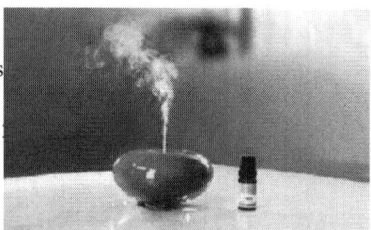

great during the Spring and Summer months. Keep inhaling this blend it will do wonders for your immune system in helping give it a boost!

18. Citrus Mist Blend
Ingredients:

- three drops of Lime
- three drops of Lemon
- two drops of Wild Orange
- two drops of Grapefruit
- one drop of Bergamot

Instructions:

This nice blend will give your home environment a lovely aroma of clean and happy—is that not what we all want are homes to smell like?

19. Breath Better Blend
Ingredients:

- two drops of Lime
- two drops of Lemon
- two drops of Peppermint
- one drop of Eucalyptus
- one drop of Rosemary

Instructions:

You are going to find once you have used this blend you will feel that it is easier for you to breathe. There is nothing worse when you are having trouble breathing.

20. Bedtime Blend
Ingredients:

- one drop of Ylang Ylang
- one drop of Bergamot
- three drops of Lavender
- two drops of Patchouli

Instructions:

Diffuse this oil blend in your bedroom half an hour before you are ready to go to sleep. Then, snuggle down in bed and get ready to have a pleasant night's sleep.

21. The Guys Blend
Ingredients:

- four drops of White Fir
- one drop of Cypress EO
- two drops of Wintergreen

Instructions:

This is a great blend for the guys out there—this is a wonderful masculine kind of aroma that you will love! It will make your man cave smell awesome!

22. Stop and Sniff the Flowery Blend
Ingredients:

- two drops of Geranium
- two drops of Clary Sage
- one drop of Lavender
- one drop of Roman Chamomile

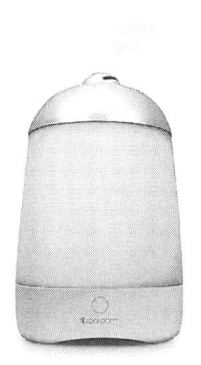

Instructions:

When you inhale this wonderful blend you are going to feel that you are sitting in the middle of a giant bouquet of flowers!

23. Joyful Blend
Ingredients:

- five drops of Wild Orange
- three drops of White Fir
- four drops of Geranium
- four drops of Bergamot

Instructions:

You will feel your mood change to one of joy and contentment when you inhale this lovely blend of oils.

24. Keep Those Nasty Bugs Away Blend
Ingredients:

- five drops of Lemongrass
- one drop of Melaleuca
- one drop of Thyme
- three drops of Eucalyptus
- two drops of Rosemary

Instructions:

Keep the pesky bugs away with this great natural bug repellant, diffuse this blend and the bugs will flee.

25. Nite Nite Blend
Ingredients:

- six drops of Vetiver
- twenty-five drops of Lavender

Instructions:

This is a great blend that is going to have you finding a restful night. Blend these oils with some fractionated coconut oil and put into a roller bottle and apply before you are ready to sleep. You will be heading to dreamland in no time!

26. Getting A Boost Blend
Ingredients:

- six drops of Peppermint
- six drops of Wild Orange

Instructions:

When you blend this up and diffuse you are suddenly going to find that you have a boost of energy!

27. Peaceful Bliss Blend
Ingredients:

- three drops of Lavender
- two drops of Sweet Marjoram
- two drops of Chamomile
- two drops of Ylang Ylang
- three drops of Vanilla Extract

Instructions:

After you have diffused this blend you can now relax and inhale a whole lot of Peace and contentment!

28. Looking Lively Blend
Ingredients:

- two drops of Lemongrass
- two drops of Wild Orange
- two drops of Grapefruit
- two drops of Tangerine
- two drops of Bergamot
- two drops of Vanilla Absolute

Instructions:

Inhale this blend and feel yourself become energized and looking lively!

29. Cheery Breaths Blend
Ingredients:

- one drop of lime
- four drops of Wintergreen
- three drops of White Fir
- three drops of Cypress

Instructions:

With this wonderful blend once you diffuse them you are going to feel yourself being lifted in spirits to a cheery state of mind!

30. The Healing Blend
Ingredients:

- three drops of Wild Orange
- three drops of Bergamot
- two drops of lemon
- two drops of Frankincense

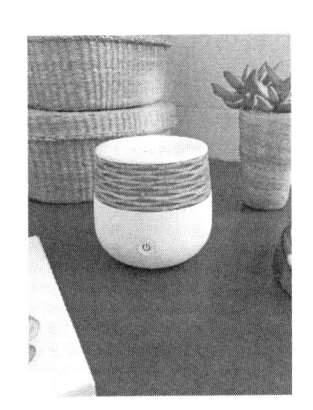

Instructions:

After you have diffused you oils you can begin your healing process, you will feel better in no time.

31. Relaxed Breathing Blend
Ingredients:

- three drops of Breathe
- three drops of Eucalyptus
- three drops of Peppermint

Instructions:

Blend your oils and diffuse them and you will find that you are going to be breathing with more ease after inhaling this blend of oils.

32. Leaving the Worry Behind Blend
- five drops of Lavender
- four drops of Clary Sage
- three drops of Ylang Ylang
- three drops Marjoram

Directions:

Blend and diffuse these oils and they will give you that extra lift you need to do your exercise workout.

33. Exercise Boost Blend
Ingredients:
- four drops of Slim and Sassy
- four drops of Peppermint
- four drops of Grapefruit
- two drops of lemon

Instructions:

This is a great blend of oils to diffuse on that day when you are feeling you don't have the energy to do your physical workout. Once you have inhaled this blend you will be ready to jump into your exercise!

34. Feeling Frisky Blend
Ingredients:

- five drops of Cassia
- five drops of Wild Orange

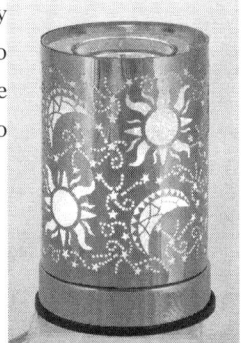

Instructions:

With this wonderful blend of oils you will find yourself feeling a bit frisky—good for a night of romance! You might say that romance is in the air!

35. Tuned In Blend
Ingredients:

- five drops of Frankincense
- four drops of Vetiver
- three drops of Balance

Instructions:

At times when you really need to stay in tune and keep yourself focused this is a great blend that will help you do just that!

36. Calm Blend
Ingredients:

- ten drops of Chamomile
- ten drops of Wild Orange
- twenty drops of Marjoram
- twenty drops of Lavender

Instructions:

You will find that your home will feel like a nice and calm place, allowing you to relax and enjoy this nice blend of oils that calms your home atmosphere.

37. Keeping Allergies at Bay Blend
Ingredients:

- three drops of Peppermint
- four drops of Lavender
- four drops of Lemon

Instructions:

Enjoy the feeling of having no allergy irritations bothering you when you diffuse this blend of oils. Say goodbye to watering eyes and stuffy noses.

38. Citrus Garden Blend
Ingredients:

- three drops of Wild Orange
- three drops of Tangerine
- three drops of Lemon
- three drops of Lime
- three drops of Bergamot

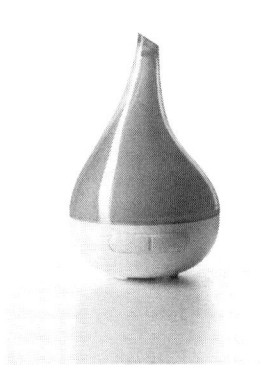

Instructions:

You will enjoy the lovely smell of citrus floating through your home with this lovely blend of citrus oils.

39. A Little Ray of Sunshine Blend
Ingredients:

- three drops of Grapefruit
- three drops of Wild Orange
- three drops of Bergamot
- three drops of Lime

Instructions:

Diffuse this blend and feel that you are in a sunny yard with fresh oranges hanging on the trees!

40. Easy Breathing Blend
Ingredients:

- one drop of Lime
- one drop of Lemon
- three drops of Peppermint
- two drops of Eucalyptus

Instructions:

With this great blend you can diffuse this and find that your breathing will become less labored.

Conclusion

I hope that you will find my collection of essential oil diffuser recipes beneficial to you in helping boost your health and wellness. Look forward to feeling some great calm and peace in your hectic life when you diffuse these therapeutic oils they will make your day become a whole lot sweeter! Imagine how nice it will be for you to try this collection of blends out and get some wonderful comfort from them in different areas of your well-being. Treat yourself and your loved ones to a wonderful experience of inhaling these blends that will offer you a great way to experience essential oils aromatherapy—in the privacy of your own home. Sit back and breath in the health and wellness in the air once you have diffused!

Printed in Poland
by Amazon Fulfillment
Poland Sp. z o.o., Wrocław